Content

WHAT IS FIBER FUELED DIET

The diet helps you to get a healthy gut microbiome. It is a plant-based diet high in fiber and includes a variety of vegetables every week.

FERMENTED RECIPES

It is good to consume something fermented every day.
Fermentation makes healthy bacterias, yeasts, and fungi that act as
a probiotic for your gut.

All these can be bought in stores, but you save a big penny by making them yourself.

Prep Time: 30 minutes

Cook Time: 4 days

Total Time: 72 hours 30 minutes

Yield: 8 cups

Category: fermented, sides, preserved

Method: fermented

Cuisine: Korean

Diet: Vegan

Description

A quick and easy recipe for authentic Kimchi, full of healthy probiotics that will keep for months in the fridge. Easy, flavorful and adaptable! Vegan adaptable!

Ingredients

2 pounds napa cabbage, cored and cut into 1-inch pieces (one large cabbage)

¼ cup sea salt (60 grams)

2 cups daikon radish, cut into matchstick strips (optional, or use carrots)

1 bunch scallions, trimmed and cut into 1-inch pieces

1 tablespoon fresh ginger, sliced (2-3 disks, peels ok)

6 cloves garlic, whole

1 shallot, quartered (optional)

2–6 tablespoons Korean-style red pepper flakes (gochugaru) or sub gochujang – see notes!

2 tablespoons fish sauce (or use vegan fish sauce, shrimp paste, miso paste, or soy sauce), more to taste

2 teaspoons sugar (or an alternative like honey, brown rice syrup)

OPTIONAL:1 tablespoon glutenous rice powder (see notes)

Instructions

SALT THE CABBAGE (6-8 hours): Reserve 1-2 outer leaves of the napa cabbage and refrigerate for later use (wrap in plastic). Cut the remaining cabbage and place it in a large bowl with the salt and toss. Add enough cool water to cover the cabbage and stir until salt is dissolved. Keep the cabbage submerged with a plate over the bowl and let stand at room temperature 6-8 hours (giving a stir midway through if possible) or overnight.

Drain the cabbage, saving the brine. Rinse the cabbage (not excessively, just a little quick rinse), drain, squeeze out any excess water, or blot with paper towels, and place it back in the bowl, adding the daikon radish and scallions.

Make the PASTE: Place the ginger, garlic, shallot, red pepper flakes, fish sauce (or alternatives) and sugar in your food processor. Add optional rice powder (see notes!) Process until well combined, pulsing, until it becomes a thick paste.

MASSAGE: Scoop the paste over the cabbage and using tongs or gloves, mix and massage the vegetables and the red pepper mixture together really well, until well coated.

PACK the cabbage into a large, two-quart jar (or two, quart jars) or a crock, leaving 1-2 inches room at the top for juices to release. Add a little of the reserved brine to just cover the vegetables, pressing them down a bit (so they are submerged) Place the whole cabbage leaf over top, pressing down- this should help keep the kimchi submerged under the brine. You can also use a fermentation weight placed over top of the whole leaf to keep it submerged. Or a small zip lock filled with water. Basically anything that touches air may mold – but no worries if this happens (see notes) it is not ruined.

 FERMENT (3-4 days) Cover loosely with a lid (allowing air to escape) and place the jar in a baking dish (or big bowl) to collect any juices that may escape. (The idea though, is to keep as much of the flavorful juice in the jar, so don't overfill.) Leave this somewhere dark and cool (55F-65F is ideal) for 3 days. A basement or lower cooler cabinet in the pantry or kitchen away from appliances works best.

EVENING OF DAY 3: Check for fermentation action or bubbles. Tap the jar and see if tiny bubbles rise to the top. Check for overflow (which also indicates fermentation). If you see bubbles, it is ready to store in the refrigerator where it will continue to ferment and develop more flavor slowly. For a softer tangier kimchi, you can continue to ferment for 3 more days or longer. If no action, give it another day or two. If you don't see bubbles when tapping the jar, it just may need a couple more days- especially in cooler climates. Be patient. See the troubleshooting section below.

REFRIGERATE: After you see bubbles (usually 3-5 days) the kimchi is ready, but it won't achieve its full flavor and complexity, until about 2 weeks (in the fridge) slowly fermenting. The longer you ferment, the more complex and tangy the taste. If you like a fizzy brine, tighten the lid, burping every week or so. If you don't want to think about it, give the lid one loose twist, so it's on there, but gases can escape.

Maintenance: This will keep for months on end in the fridge (as long as it is submerged in the brine) and will continue to ferment very slowly, getting more and more flavorful. Feel free to remove the cabbage leaf and just press kimchi down under the brine, after each use. (See notes for adding more brine.)

SERVE: Serve it as side dish: scoop it out using a slotted spoon, place in a small bowl, drizzle with sesame oil , toasted sesame seeds, and fresh scallions. Or Use it in Kimchi Fried Rice, Kimchi Burritos, Seoul Bowls, Kimchi Soup!

2. Sauerkraut is probably the

most well-known lacto-fermented vegetable. Old fashioned sauerkraut is made with thinly sliced cabbage and salt. Like any traditionally homemade food, sauerkraut can be made in a number of ways with a number of ingredients. Whether you add a secret ingredient to your homemade sauerkraut or keep it basic, kraut has a slew of health benefits. It is rich in probiotics, vitamins, fiber, and minerals, which can contribute to better digestion and a stronger immune system. Sauerkraut can also help promote a healthy heart, stronger bones, and weight loss.

Even if each kraut-making method is different there are a few common basics to remember when making fermented cabbage into sauerkraut at home.

EASY TIPS FOR MAKING GOOD SAUERKRAUT

Use fresh cabbage. The better your ingredients, the better the finished product will be.

Use at least some salt. Salt is a traditional ingredient in sauerkraut because it increases shelf life, texture, and flavor. The amount of salt used can vary according to personal taste preference. We recommend 1 to 3 Tbsp. per quart of water. When making sauerkraut, it's also important to choose the right salt, like Celtic Sea Salt. For those that don't want to use salt, check out our salt-free sauerkraut recipe.

Create an anaerobic environment. This is an absolute essential step in the sauerkraut-making process. The cabbage must be completely submerged underneath a brine in order for the lactic acid bacteria to proliferate. This is important for protecting your lactic acid fermentation from unwanted bacteria (or mold). Fermentation weights can help keep your cabbage submerged.

Give it time. You can ferment sauerkraut for only a few days before moving to cold storage, but giving sauerkraut a lower temperature and longer fermentation time can develop the flavor and texture a little better. We suggest letting it ferment for 2 weeks, though experimenting with time and taste is the best way to determine what time frame works best for you.

Need more tips? Take a look at how to ferment vegetables and when to place them in cold storage.

SUPPLIES FOR MAKING SAUERKRAUT

When it comes to fermentation supplies, there are a lot of tools out there to choose from, each claiming to be the best solution for perfectly fermented kraut. This can be a bit overwhelming you're new to making fermented foods, and just trying to figure what you need to get started.

RECIPE: HOMEMADE SAUERKRAUT

Homemade Sauerkraut

Sauerkraut is probably the most well-known lacto-fermented vegetable. Old fashioned sauerkraut is made with thinly sliced cabbage and salt. Like any traditionally homemade food, sauerkraut can be made in a number of ways with a number of ingredients. Whether you add a secret ingredient to your homemade sauerkraut or keep it basic, kraut has a slew of health benefits. It is rich in probiotics, vitamins, fiber, and minerals, which can contribute to better digestion and a stronger immune system. Sauerkraut can also help promote a healthy heart, stronger bones, and weight loss.

Even if each kraut-making method is different there are a few common basics to remember when making fermented cabbage into sauerkraut at home.

START MAKING HOMEMADE SAUERKRAUT NOW!

sauerkraut kit homemade

Homemade Sauerkraut Kit

EASY TIPS FOR MAKING GOOD SAUERKRAUT

Use fresh cabbage. The better your ingredients, the better the finished product will be.

Use at least some salt. Salt is a traditional ingredient in sauerkraut because it increases shelf life, texture, and flavor. The amount of salt used can vary according to personal taste preference. We recommend 1 to 3 Tbsp. per quart of water. When making sauerkraut, it's also important to choose the right salt, like Celtic Sea Salt. For those that don't want to use salt, check out our salt-free sauerkraut recipe.

Create an anaerobic environment. This is an absolute essential step in the sauerkraut-making process. The cabbage must be completely submerged underneath a brine in order for the lactic acid bacteria to proliferate. This is important for protecting your lactic acid fermentation from unwanted bacteria (or mold). Fermentation weights can help keep your cabbage submerged.

Give it time. You can ferment sauerkraut for only a few days before moving to cold storage, but giving sauerkraut a lower temperature and longer fermentation time can develop the flavor and texture a little better. We suggest letting it ferment for 2 weeks, though experimenting with time and taste is the best way to determine what time frame works best for you.

Need more tips? Take a look at how to ferment vegetables and when to place them in cold storage.

SUPPLIES FOR MAKING SAUERKRAUT

When it comes to fermentation supplies, there are a lot of tools out there to choose from, each claiming to be the best solution for perfectly fermented kraut. This can be a bit overwhelming you're new to making fermented foods, and just trying to figure what you need to get started.

Our tutorial Fermentation Equipment: Choosing the Right Supplies goes into detail about different options, but the reality is having the basics like a good knife, container for fermenting, a fermentation weight, and some sort of lid with an airlock is all you need to get started.

METHODS FOR MAKING SAUERKRAUT

1. SLICING, POUNDING, AND KNEADING CABBAGE

Thinly slice cabbage, salt it, then pound it with a tool such as the Cabbage Crusher or Pickle Packer for about 10 minutes, or until enough juice is released to form a brine and completely cover the cabbage.

Move the cabbage and juice to fermentation containers, weigh the cabbage down to keep it below the brine. Cover with tight-fitting lids, airlock lids, or a tight-weave cloth, secured with a rubber band.

2. WEIGHTING AND PRESSING KRAUT IN A CROCK

Place shredded cabbage and salt in a large fermentation crock or bowl. Instead of pounding, weigh the cabbage down with heavy bowls or pebbles. Press on the weights regularly to draw the natural juices out of the cabbage and submerge the cabbage slowly in the brine.

After a couple of days, with continued pressing, the cabbage will have accumulated a fair amount of liquid at the top, enough to cover the cabbage completely.

3. WHOLE CABBAGE HEADS WITH BRINE

In this method, the cabbage is not shredded or sliced prior to fermenting. Since whole cabbage heads cannot form their own brine fast enough to protect them from mold and unwanted yeasts a brine is generally created then used for fermenting.

While this method is the least labor-intensive, it takes the longest. Four weeks or more are necessary before moving to cold storage because of the size of the cabbage heads.

HOMEMADE SAUERKRAUT AT YOUR FINGERTIPS

The easiest way to start making sauerkraut is with our Homemade Sauerkraut Kit!

This kit includes everything you need to start fermenting at home and comes with detailed instructions crafted by our fermentation experts to make everything as easy and as fun as possible.

HOMEMADE SAUERKRAUT RECIPE

Below you'll find our basic sauerkraut recipe. This recipe utilizes the pounding and kneading method. It is a great place to start for anyone just beginning to explore fermented vegetables.

Once you've mastered the basics, you can vary this recipe by adding other vegetables, herbs, and spices. Or use one of our other sauerkraut recipes for inspiration.

INGREDIENTS:

1 Medium Head of Cabbage

1-3 Tbsp. sea salt

INSTRUCTIONS:

Chop or shred cabbage. Sprinkle with salt.

Knead the cabbage with clean hands, or pound with a potato masher or Cabbage Crusher about 10 minutes, until there is enough liquid to cover.

Stuff the cabbage into a quart jar, pressing the cabbage underneath the liquid. If necessary, add a bit of water to completely cover cabbage.

Cover the jar with a tight lid, airlock lid, or coffee filter secured with a rubber band.

Culture at room temperature (60-70°F is preferred) for at least 2 weeks until desired flavor and texture are achieved. If using a tight lid, burp daily to release excess pressure.

Once the sauerkraut is finished, put a tight lid on the jar and move to cold storage. The sauerkraut's flavor will continue to develop as it ages.

VARIATIONS:

For a more complex flavor add caraway seeds (to taste).

Prior to culturing, you can also mix 1 part other vegetables or ingredients (shredded carrots, apples, etc.) with 5 parts cabbage to vary the recipe. For a non-traditional sauerkraut, try this carrot sauerkraut recipe

Pineapple Kombucha Recipe

Ingredients

3 litres of plain kombucha, freshly prepared (recipe above)

400 ml pineapple juice

Preparation

Mix the kombucha and pineapple juice.

Taste, then add more pineapple juice as needed.

Bottle the kombucha (as described in How to Bottle My Kombucha, above).

making cherry water kefir

After you've made basic water kefir a few times, it's fun to experiment with new flavors. You can flavor your basic brew with sweetened herbal teas, fruit juices or fruits like cherries.

Cherry water kefir relies on a process called secondary fermentation. That is, after you brew your initial batch, you can strain and store the tibicos grains, and ferment the water kefir a second time.

For the secondary fermentation, you'll want to use flip-top bottles. That's because these bottles will capture the carbon dioxide that builds up during fermentation. As a result, your cherry water kefir will be naturally fizzy and bubbly

making cherry water kefir

After you've made basic water kefir a few times, it's fun to experiment with new flavors. You can flavor your basic brew with sweetened herbal teas, fruit juices or fruits like cherries.

Cherry water kefir relies on a process called secondary fermentation. That is, after you brew your initial batch, you can strain and store the tibicos grains, and ferment the water kefir a second time.

For the secondary fermentation, you'll want to use flip-top bottles. That's because these bottles will capture the carbon dioxide that builds up during fermentation. As a result, your cherry water kefir will be naturally fizzy and bubbly

FIBER SMOOTHIE CUBES

This was such a fun idea from Jen Hansard. Such a simple way to meal prep smoothies and especially fiber into your diet. You make a mix of chia, hemp, psyllium husk, dates, cacao, and some liquid and pour it into ice cube trays.

I tried these without the cacao, since I think this way the tastes go well with all kinds of flavors. I added some apple puree to my cubes.

When you make your smoothie just add 1-4 fiber bombs in it.

One cube has:

Calories 70

Fiber 2,7g

Carbs 8g

Protein 2,5g

Fat 3,9g

HOW TO MAKE HIGH FIBER SMOOTHIES AND THE BEST RECIPES

Smoothies are an easy way to get fiber and phytonutrients. You can get your whole family to eat veggies and fruits in the form of smoothies.

Many people get only 15-20 grams of fiber a day. The minimum recommendations are 25 grams for women and 38 for men. I do recommend though higher intake. I personally try to get 40 grams a day. A general guideline is to get 14 grams of fiber per 1000 calories you eat. This is the minimum.

WHAT CAN YOU ADD TO YOUR SMOOTHIE TO GET FIBER

All plants have fiber, fruits, berries, spinach, kale, and seeds are a great fiber source for smoothies. Some fruits and veggies have more fiber than others. Here is a list of high fiber ingredients I recommend using for smoothies. List of fruits are further down.

Food item Fiber in grams/50 g

Kale 3,4

Broccoli 1,8

Avocado 3,4

Chia seeds 17,2

Rolled oats 5

Dates 3,6

Raspberries 1,9

Blueberries 1,6

Strawberries 0,9

Dried figs 4,7

To make your smoothie taste good, it needs some sweetness. If you want to add greens, it is good to pair them with some fruits. Dates are a great fruit that works as sweeteners; dates also have fiber in themselves. 2-3 soft dates often give smoothies enough sweetness so that your kids love them as well. Banana, mango, pear, and apple are also common fruits for sweetening.

ARE FRUIT SMOOTHIES HIGH IN FIBER?

By choosing high-fiber fruits, you can maximize your fiber intake. The highest fiber fruits are passionfruit, avocado, pomegranate, and pear. Adding 1 tablespoon of chia or flax seeds or some oats increases the fiber amount by 3 grams.

Here is a list of fiber content in some fruits that go well in smoothies and make them sweet and delicious.

Fruit/peeled, without stones Fiber in grams /100 g

Pear 3,1

Kiwi 3

Banana 2,6

Apple 2,4

Avocado 7

Persimon 3,6

Orange 2,4

Papaya 1,7

Pineapple 1,4

Cherries 1,5

Apricots 1,9

Mango 1,6

Peaches 2,1

Plums 1,7

Watermelon 1,1

Bananas are often the fruit to use to get sweetness, creaminess, and thickness for a smoothie. If you are not banana fan mangoes are a great replacement. They also give some creamy consistency. Coconut cream is the ultimate creaminess giver.

GET EXTRA FIBER FROM SEEDS

Flax seeds, chia seeds or hemp hearts are a great addition to your smoothie.

Flax seeds 1 tablespoon, 2,6 grams fiber.

Chia seeds 1 tablespoon, 3,4grams of fiber

Hemp hearts 1 tablespoon, 2,8 grams of fiber

Hemp heats , peeled, 0,4 grams of fiber

Seeds are a nutrient bomb; they have proteins, omega 3 fatty acids, antioxidants, vitamins, and minerals. Seeds are a good source of iron, calcium, magnesium, and zinc. Seeds are a good source of healthy fats that don't contain any cholesterol. Flaxseeds contain lignan, and this can help to prevent some cancers.

With seeds, it is good to limit them somewhat, since they have phytic acids. This is an antinutrient that can reduce the absorption of Iron and Zinc. Flax seeds in some areas also can have cadmium, so limiting the intake to 1 tablespoon is good. In another study, the safe limit was 50 grams a day.

TOP WITH GREENS TO BOOST WITH FIBER AND PHYTONUTRIENTS

I think greens are a must to add in your smoothie. Sometimes t can feel hard to get enough greens and you might think if it is that necessary. They are so easy to add in the smoothie and you get a lot of vitamins if you add some. Just a couple of kale leaves(30 grams) gives you 35% of vitamin A and 30% vitamin C-need that you need a day.

Greens you can add to your smoothie

Kale

Spinach

Broccoli

Celery

Mint

Collard greens

Carrot tops

Swiss chard

Bok choy

Watercress gives a spicy flavor.

Spinach is the one mildest and often kid approved also, it does not taste is you add some fruit aswell. I buy spinach as frozen, it comes handy in small cubes in the freezer bag, and it is so simple just to toss 1-2 cubes to the blender. This also makes the smoothie nice cold and refreshing.

It is also easy to add some green powders like chorella, spirulina, nettle or wheat grass powder. Remember to start with small doses since they are quite powerful and can give you for example headache or diarrhea.

ADD GRAINS TO YOUR SMOOTHIE

Some grains can be an addition of fiber to your smoothies. Oats and quinoa are for example high in soluble fiber. Rolled oats you can add directly to your smoothie. Other grains are best as cooked. Add a maximum of ½ cup grains to a big smoothie, otherwise they might take over tastewise. I like to add 2-3 tablespoons of oats in my smoothies.

Grains 50 grams The total fiber in grams

Rolled oats 5

Cooked quinoa 1,5

Amaranth flakes 3,4

Cooked barley 0,9

BENEFITS OF FIBER

Regulates bowel movements

Helps to stabilize blood glucose levels

Helps to prevent cancers

Lowers cholesterol

Helps to feel satiated

Helps to maintain a healthy weight

Does blending destroy fiber?

Blending does chop up the fiber smaller. This results in a bit faster absorption of the sugars in the smoothie.

Is it healthy to have a smoothie every day?

A non sugary smoothie with greens and fruits is great to have every day. Don´t overconsume high oxalate foods every day though, otherwise you can get kidney stones.

SUPPLEMENTS YOU CAN ADD TO YOUR SMOOTHIE FOR FIBER

Psyllium husk is one fiber type you can safely add to smoothie. One common brand name for it is metamucil.

Oat fiber is also common. Oat brans or other grain brans are a great addition to get fiber.

HIGH FIBER SMOOTHIE RECIPES

BANANA-RASPBERRY-KIWI SMOOTHIE

This recipe has 10,2 grams of fiber! You also get all the vitamin C you need for the day. All of these fruits are ones that have a high fiber content so you get naturally lots of fiber. This is also topped with some additional chia seeds. To get a nice summer drink you can use a frozen banana instead of ice.

Calories 230

Fiber 10,2g

Carbs 43g

Protein 4g

Fat 3g

Healthy Oil-Free Granol

Description

The best Healthy Oil-Free Granola recipe! It's simple to make, sweetened with maple syrup, crunchy, and super delicious. Serve in a bowl with your favorite plant milk for a delicious breakfast or enjoy all by itself as a snack.

Ingredients

SCALE

1X

2X

3X

4 cups old-fashioned rolled oats

½ cup steel-cut oats (optional)

1 cup chopped walnuts

¼ cup flaxseed meal

2 tsp. ground cinnamon

½ cup pure maple syrup

½ cup unsweetened applesauce

1 Tbsp vanilla extract

Instructions

Preheat oven to 350°F and line a baking sheet with parchment paper.

Put all the dry ingredients into a large bowl and mix everything together.

Pour the wet ingredients evenly over the dry oat mixture and toss until everything is well covered and combined.

Spread the granola evenly over the baking sheet and bake for 35-40 minutes until its golden. But, be careful not to let it burn. Gently toss the granola halfway through the cooking process.

Once the granola is done baking remove it from the oven let it cool for 15-20 minutes.

www.ingramcontent.com/pod-product-compliance
Lightning Source LLC
Chambersburg PA
CBHW051928250726

48659CB00002B/904